THE SECRET TO LOOKING LIKE YOU

The Latest European Injection Techniques from a Belarusian Dermatologist.

BY MARINA VASHKEVICH

ISBN: 978-1-9992565-0-0

REGISTER & CLAIM YOUR GIFTS!

- Free Consultation
- $25 Gift Card to be applied toward any treatment of choice

Visit www.MedVSpa.com to register!

TABLE OF CONTENTS

REGISTER & CLAIM YOUR GIFTS! 3

INTRODUCTION 7

CHAPTER 1: LOOKING IN THE MIRROR 9

Are Beauty Injections a Necessity? 10

CHAPTER 2: STRUCTURAL AND TISSUE AGING 13

How Does Your Face Age? 14

CHAPTER 3: FACE HARMONY 17

Do You Need to Pay Attention to the Symmetry? .. 18

CHAPTER 4: THE CAUSE OF PERMANENT WRINKLES 21

How Does Your Muscle Movement Affect Your Aging?
.... 22

CHAPTER 5: INDICATIONS FOR INJECTIONS 25

When Should I Start Doing Injections? 26

CHAPTER 6: LET'S GET REAL 31

What Product do You Need? The Difference Between
Botulinum Toxin, Fillers and Mesotherapy 32

CHAPTER 7: LET'S ASSESS YOUR AGING SIGNS............ 37

How Old Do You Actually Look? 38

CHAPTER 8: DOUBLE CHIN AND JAWLINE 47

Reversing Time in the Lower Third of the Face 48

CHAPTER 9: THE NATURAL LOOK 53

Why are Some People Overdone? 54

CHAPTER 10: THE LONG-TERM GOALS 59

How Often Should I Have Injections?....................... 60

CHAPTER 11: YOUR FACE'S SAFETY 63

What are the Criteria for Facial Injections? 64

CHAPTER 12: START FROM THE CONSULTATION 67

What Can You Expect? 68

CHAPTER 13: THE INJECTION CARD 71

What Your Injector Needs to Know........................... 72

CHAPTER 14: TREATMENT OF AGING ON THE FOREHEAD 75

What Botulinum Toxin can do for the Forehead 76

CHAPTER 15: THE HATED "ELEVENTH"............................. 77

How do You Get Rid of the Frown Lines?............... 78

CHAPTER 16: AN EYE OPENER 85

Open Eyes and Eyebrow Lifting with Injections 86

CHAPTER 17: LIPS – THE MOST "FEARFUL" AREA......... 91

Why You Can't Look Complete without Lip Fillers 92

CHAPTER 18: AFTERWORD.. 99

Why This Matters 100

REFERENCES 103

ABOUT THE AUTHOR 104

INTRODUCTION

I have many clients whose husbands complain they're becoming older and older, whereas their wives are becoming younger and younger. What is the secret of such transformation? Are beauty injections the only solution to looking better? Are they a non-avoidable necessity to look younger? Do you know how many units of Botox you need and how much fillers will keep your look natural? This book has been created with the idea of clarifying the field of beauty injections for ordinary people. The injections world is growing, and every day in my practice, I see more and more people who either have done injections, are looking for injections to be done, or who absolutely deny injections. Some people really feel lost in this field.

For me, aesthetic dermatology is like an open book. Originally, I got my MD in Belarus, so I'm a certified Belarusian dermatologist as well as a Canadian and American registered nurse. I have clinics with the same sets of the equipment, and we use the same unique combination of technologies and injections in Belarus and in Canada.

My goal is to help regular customers understand how many injections they need, what is the best time for them to start, and how often filler injections, Botulinum Toxin (Botox, Dysport) and Mesotherapy (Bio- Revitalization) should be repeated. Moreover, it's simple to use the information provided in this book to understand the world of injections. Let me clarify this field for you.

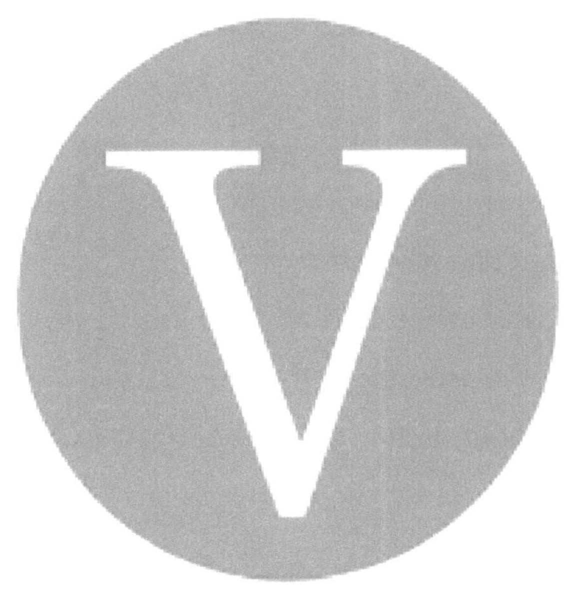

CHAPTER 1:
LOOKING
IN THE MIRROR

Are Beauty Injections a Necessity?

If you opened this book, you are probably starting to notice more severe signs of aging, or perhaps, only the first little bit of time has started showing on your face. Either way, when you look closely in the mirror do you perhaps notice crow's feet around your eyes, creasing wrinkles on your forehead, deeper under-eye circles that never seem to go away, permanent smile lines, and a less defined jawline? Has your face been looking wrinklier and saggier than you remember? Did you stop liking yourself in pictures because of a double chin appearance? Don't be frightened by these changes. I may just have a solution to help you quickly and effectively. And best of all, this solution will keep you looking natural while allowing you to return your youth. The result everyone wants is a fresher looking face with less aggravated aging features that makes them confident in the way they look. They want to love the way they look in the mirror first thing in the morning. No one wants a plasticky, unmoving face that looks like a stretched canvas. What feels right is returning your face to the way it used to be 10 or even 20 years ago. These goals can be reached via three different methods that don't require surgery or a prolonged recovery period. They all do, however, give immediate and wonderful results.

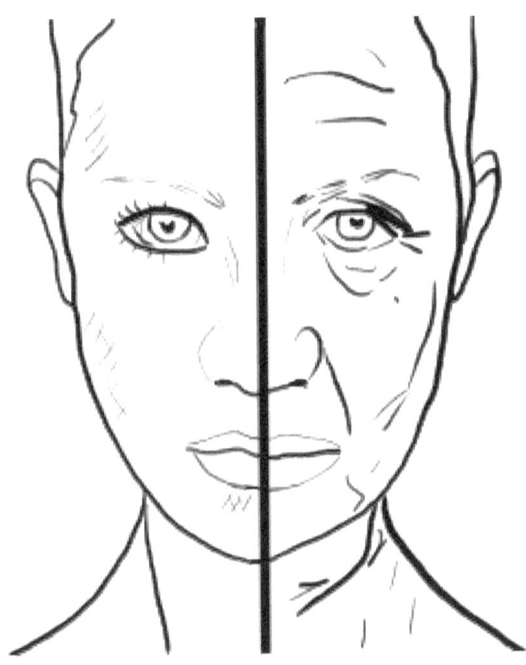

In this book, my goal is to walk you through how these methods work, why they are effective, and which one would be suitable for your needs specifically. Your life can change just like the lives of thousands of other women who turned to injections to restore their youth.

These three methods have changed the appearances and lives of many others, and your life could be next.

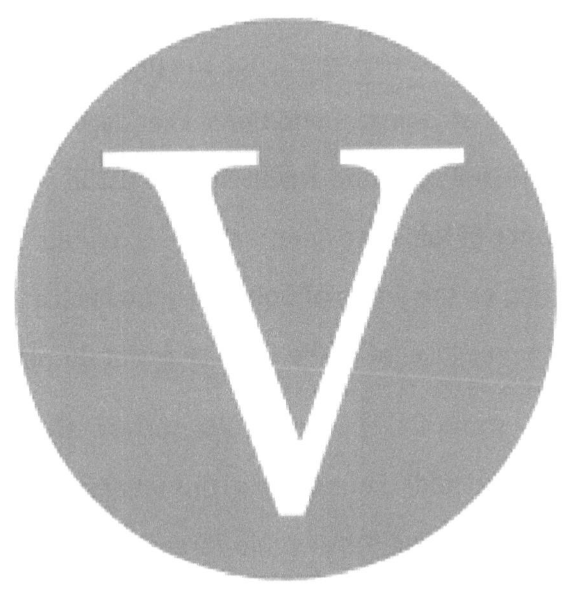

CHAPTER 2:
STRUCTURAL AND
TISSUE AGING

How Does Your Face Age?

As we grow older, we experience the processes of tissue and structural aging. Conditions like dark spots, big pores, and dull skin tone are all signs of tissue aging. The appearance of folds and deep wrinkles is related to structural aging on the levels of bone-fat-muscles (Le Louarn, 2007). People lose fat in the deep layers of the skin.

However, some fat appears in the surface of the face, creating deep folds. For example, this fat appears as bags under the eyes, the malar mold (areas under the lower eyelid), nasolabial folds, jowls, and a double chin. Repeated facial muscle movements cause expelling of the gat and the appearance of hollows within the fac.

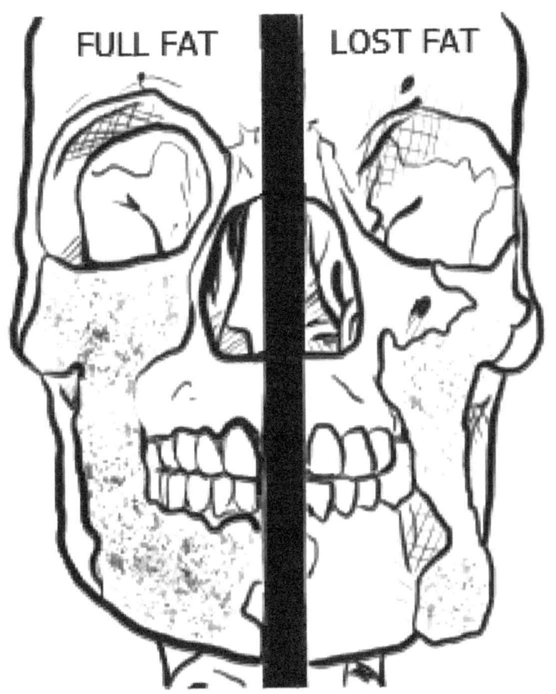

Muscles change, as well. Le Louarn thinks that muscles involved in facial expressions are becoming shorter with age, increasing their tone and losing their curvature. Muscles on young faces are convex-shaped and long while the face is relaxed. However, with age, they change shape, becoming rectilinear; the length becomes shorter upon contraction as well.

It is easily explainable that the muscles shorten and lose convexity because they are mostly in hyper tone due to aging. To handle the structural aging process, we have to use Mesotherapy, fillers, and Neurotoxin injections.

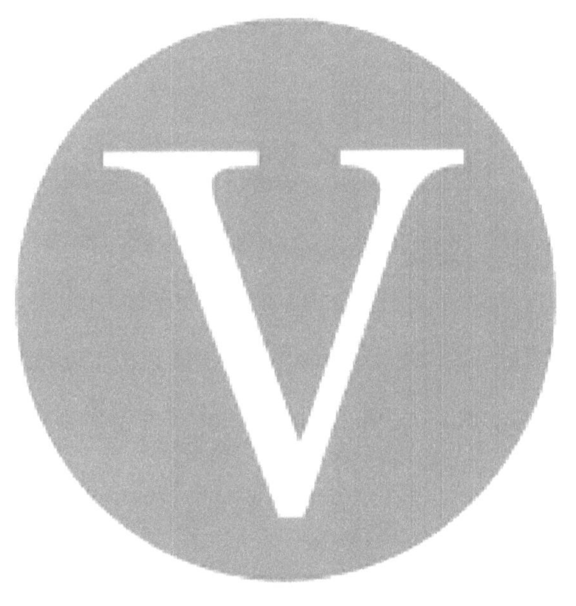

CHAPTER 3:
FACE HARMONY

Do You Need to Pay Attention to the Symmetry?

One's face is the most beautiful when changes are noticed by the client, rather than onlookers. Therefore face harmony is one of the goals of the aesthetic correction. The face should be assessed according to the criteria of symmetry and balance. The assessment includes:

1. A genetic predisposition to facial expressions; one may look at their mother's muscle behavior, which causes wrinkles like neck circles and forehead creases to determine their own potential patterns.

2. Type of muscular activity, meaning the way one may use their muscles. There are three ways to define muscular activity, including:

    a. The hyperkinetic type (often using the facial muscles to communicate aggressive expressions).

    b. The kinetic type (using the facial muscles in a common way that others do).

    c. The hypokinetic type (barely using any facial expression to convey emotion).

(De Maio, 2007)

3. Aging changes and their severity. I rarely see people who are objectively looking at themselves. Much of the population today may look at themselves subjectively rather than objectively. This is an indicator that they need professional opinions.

4. The specific face anatomy, such as a wide space between the eyebrows and muscular balance/imbalance. For instance, if one side of the lips works more than the other while you are talking or if one eyebrow is higher than the other.

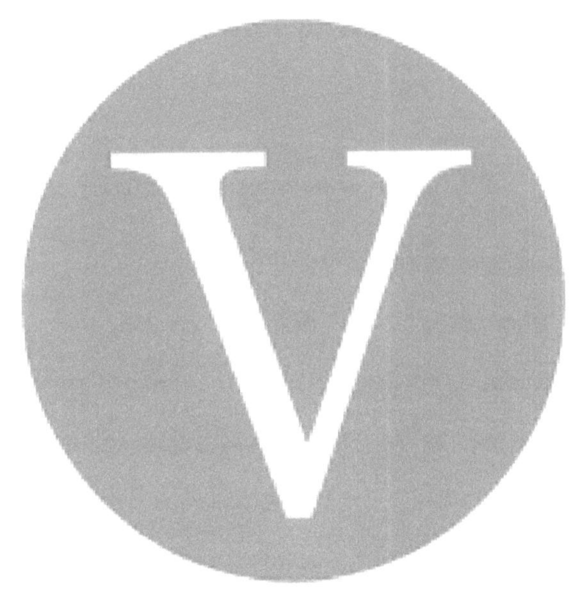

CHAPTER 4:
THE CAUSE OF
PERMANENT WRINKLES

How Does Your Muscle Movement Affect Your Aging?

How does your muscle movement affect your aging?

It is important to understand how aggressive your face muscle movements are because contracting muscles move fat pats and even bones underneath them. With age, facial muscle activity increases and leads to hyper tone (Le Louran, 2007). Therefore you may see elderly people with permanent muscle tension between the eyebrows, or near the corners of the lips. These rigid muscles press the fat below, and then the fat moves. Fat appears on the surface as nasolabial folds or jowls, and this movement is a part of the natural aging process that takes place. Therefore, it is important to understand facial muscle activity to prevent the imperfections mentioned above. Patterns of muscle activity were described by Maio M. (De Maio, 2007). He divided people into three different groups, based on the activity of their face muscles.

It is predictable, that if hyperkinetic muscle activity is not corrected, as the result of the aging process, these groups of muscles will be in a high muscle activity range. People in the hypertonic group of people show spastic type muscle contractions. They complain that they experience difficulties relaxing muscles or resting. When I take before, and after pictures, I ask clients to relax. However, many of them continuously keep a smile on their face, despite their effort to relax. This smile reflects the hyperactivity of the muscles around the mouth. Relaxing these muscles results in a younger appearance. Clients that constantly use forehead muscles to keep their eyebrows lifted have deep forehead lines. If this pattern was not broken at an early age, specialists are powerless to do anything, except surgery. However, it is easy to prevent this contractile component (active tension, produced by contraction of the muscle) (De Maio, 2019).

Some aging people express permanent surprises on their faces. This is a contractile component of the lateral part of the eyebrow muscles. If these muscles were relaxed with Botulinum toxin between the ages of 40 and 50 several times, this aging sign could be prevented. The most popular aging treatment in the world is injections of a neurotoxin. This is an especially effective treatment when the forehead shows a lot of wrinkles. Lines, which appear between your eyebrows, crow's feet around the eyes and droopy tails of the eyebrows, are conditions which can be successfully treated with neurotoxin as well. Botulinum toxin treatment gives a much younger look. It lifts the eyebrows and opens the eyes. After an injection treatment, the forehead wrinkles can completely disappear, or the injection can only lift the eyebrows, helping the face to express emotions in a softer way. Several years ago, the technic, called Nefertiti, was introduced on the market to make the jawline more defined. This substance interrupts the transmission of the impulse to the muscle. As a result, the muscle either stops responding to the impulse completely, or the response is radically decreased for 3 to 4 months.

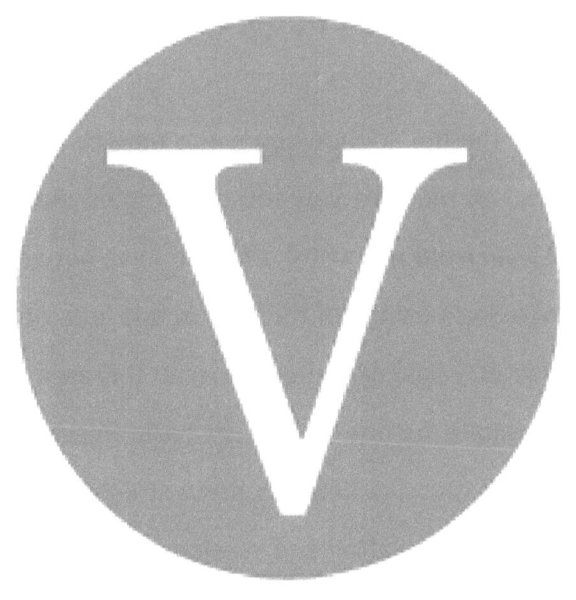

CHAPTER 5:
INDICATIONS FOR INJECTIONS

When Should I Start Doing Injections?

To answer the question, when is the time to start using injections, let me give you some examples. Recently, I saw a 29-year-old girl who hated the lines between her eyebrows. She's using her muscles in this area on a very aggressive way. Her skin shows lines in this area. She's a good candidate for the Botulinum toxin injections. The relaxation of muscles helps to prevent lines to become deeper. Moreover, after 3- 4 sessions of injections, she probably will forget how to use the muscles in this area in the strong way she is using them now.

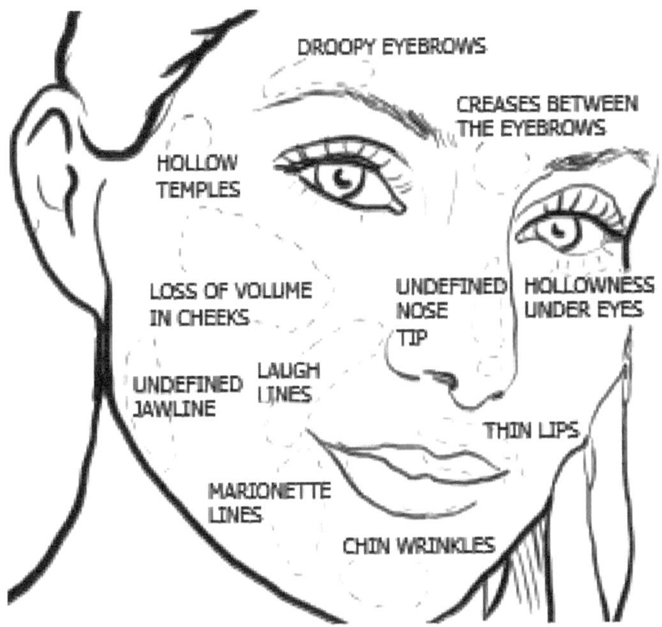

It means that she should feel free to stop doing injections in the area between the eyebrows, and she will enjoy her look without these deep lines.

Here's another example. I saw a young boy who was looking for a business career. He's frowning his forehead constantly, five times per 10 seconds, as he's talking with other people. He's a good candidate for the neurotoxin injections as well with the goal to prevent the appearance of wrinkles. A man needs a higher amount of Botulinum toxin because his muscles are stronger. After three sessions of injection, done every 3-4 months, his forehead lines will look smoother. But because he is in business, he wants his face to express emotions. Then he will be injected in such a way that his forehead will not be frozen. In expressing emotions, he will move his muscles and skin, but when he is calm, he will not see any wrinkles.

The most effective treatment to replace volume, which we're losing as a result of the aging process is filler injections. It's very easy to understand if we need fillers or not. When you see holes in your temples area, or you see holes near your ear, these are conditions which we successfully treat with filler injections.

When you look at yourself and see in the middle part of your face, a hole in the area of the cheek, it's a condition that will respond to filler injections. If you see that your lips are barely visible, this is a condition for the filler injections. In addition, many young people consider fillers to follow the trend of social media to have perfectly lifted cheekbones or prominent appealing lips.

To sum up, we use Botulinum toxin to decrease the spasm of the muscles, fillers to replace lost volume and both of them to achieve the effect of skin lifting.

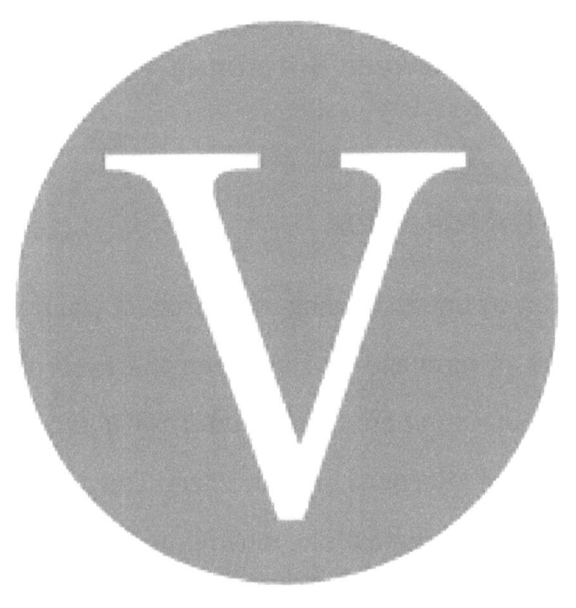

CHAPTER 6:
LET'S GET REAL

What Product do You Need? The Difference Between Botulinum Toxin, Fillers and Mesotherapy

PLACEMENT FOR BOTOX

Let's start by understanding what product you need. For the area of forehead and between the eyebrows, the most popular solution is Botulinum Toxin injections. Botulinum toxin injections are not fillers. They are used to decrease the strength of the muscles and to reach the effect of complete muscle relaxation or partial muscle relaxation. When talking about the muscle spasms, the strengths are evaluated. Please pay attention to the muscle activity, but not to the depths of your wrinkles.

So how do we assess muscle activity? Just put a finger between the eyebrows and start frowning. When you do this, you will definitely understand the strength of your muscles. Put two of your fingers over the heads of your eyebrows and frown. In this way, you are assessing the strength of another group of muscles in the area between eyebrows. All of these muscles are responsible for your " eleventh." If you found those muscles strong, consider around 20 Units of Botox. If they are not strong, you might need around 15 Units. Look at your forehead when you express surprise. If it doesn't move or moves barely, don't agree to do neurotoxin injections. But if you use those muscles a lot, do injections. Injections of Botulinum toxin in this area can be done with two goals. First, it freezes the muscles to achieve the result of an absolutely smooth forehead. The four points injections method is usually selected.

The second way injections can be done is through what's called a lifting technic. This helps to lift the forehead, saving some range of movements. There are multiple ways to receive injections. When you receive injections, you will enjoy a forehead without wrinkles when you are calm; however, you will still be able to show emotions in a very natural way. The difference between the two is the number of sites for injections.

After 50 years old, some people use their forehead naturally to lift up the eyebrows. Botulinum toxin injections will be used for this forehead lifting in a smaller dosage. This gets the eyebrows lifting but does not produce full muscle relaxation; otherwise, the risk of eyebrows dropping appears. To get this look, the dosage should be decreased by about 30-50%.

Look at your chin. Do you use it much when you're talking? Using chin muscles is an aggressive sign of aging as well. It's so easy to do one or two site injections in this area to stop the chin talking. Your perioral area will look much proportional and younger.

PLACEMENT FOR FILLERS

The most effective treatment to replace volume is filler injections. Regional fillers were developed to replace the volume which we're losing because of the aging process. It's very easy to assess if we need fillers, or not. When you see a dip in your temple area or you see a hollower space near your ear, these are the conditions which can be successfully treated with injections.

When you look at yourself and see a spot that lost volume in your cheek, this is a condition to be improved by filler injections. If you see that your lips are barely visible, this is a condition that will respond to filler injections. In addition, many young people consider fillers to follow the trend created by social media to have perfectly lifted cheekbones or prominent appealing lips.

MESOTHERAPY

Let's move forward and talk about the very popular therapy practiced in Europe called Mesotherapy. "Meso" means middle. Mesotherapy involves the injection of active ingredients into different skin layers.

Mesotherapy accomplishes several goals. One, it stimulates the growth of collagen. Two, Mesotherapy injects skin hydration deep into the skin. Goal number three is the creation of the vectors of lifting. Removal of fat from the double chin using injections can be accomplished through Mesotherapy as well. In this therapy, we stimulate our own skin to produce new collagen. After therapy, one looks very natural with lifted cheekbones and a prominent jawline. So, you would look fabulous, but very natural.

Mesotherapy is a great tool that can be started from the age of 20. Don't be surprised. We use hyaluronic acid to raise the immunity of the skin. Very often, when I see clients with acne, or when I see rosacea stage one or two, I recommend Mesotherapy. For such clients, raising skin immunity with Mesotherapy is a great solution to handle skin problems.

I have many young girls who do these injections. Mesotherapy helps them to get rid of pimples, and to make their skin look plumper and hydrated. A series of a minimum of four treatments is recommended. Numbing cream is applied before the treatment. Injections are performed around the face/ neck/décolleté in a deep skin layer.

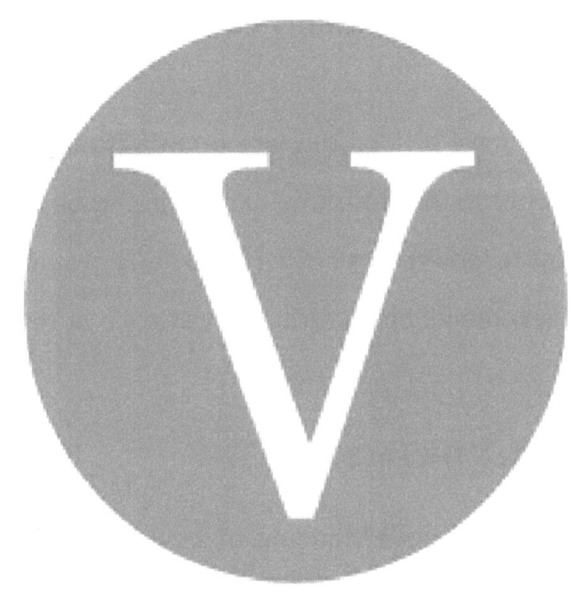

CHAPTER 7:
LET'S ASSESS
YOUR AGING SIGNS

How Old Do You Actually Look?

Specialists have divided the face up into three different parts. I offer to use this same pattern in this book to explain how to look younger using the criteria of beauty and the achievements of contemporary science at the same time.

UPPER 1/3 OF THE FACE

To give you an understanding of how much filler you need, we continue with an assessment. Let's move from the upper part of your face; starting with the temple area. Do you feel the hollows between your hairline and eyebrows? Women tend to have this cave.

However, with age, the curve becomes deeper, changing the facial shape. The face, being curved and previously shaped similarly to an oval, starts to look more angular and long. Imagine this area being refilled. Do your eyes seem more open now? Does your face, once again, seem more rejuvenated and oval-like? If the answer is yes, this area would greatly benefit from being injected with fillers. You may choose to use a 0.5-1 syringe for the left and right temple areas of the face.

MIDDLE 1/3 OF THE FACE

Many people experience fear and are opposed to injections in the middle part of the face; commonly around the cheekbone area. I completely agree that prominent and visible underlying cheekbones make people look "done," "weird," and "look like others." These injections are especially noticeable when people smile. The cheekbones may look unnaturally big, giving the illusion of smaller eyes. This area is very tricky not to over-inject. I will guide you through a controlled, step-by-step process to injecting, avoiding any problems of excess. First of all, when the product is put down in vectors, it shows a much smoother result, compared to when a certain amount is put into one spot.

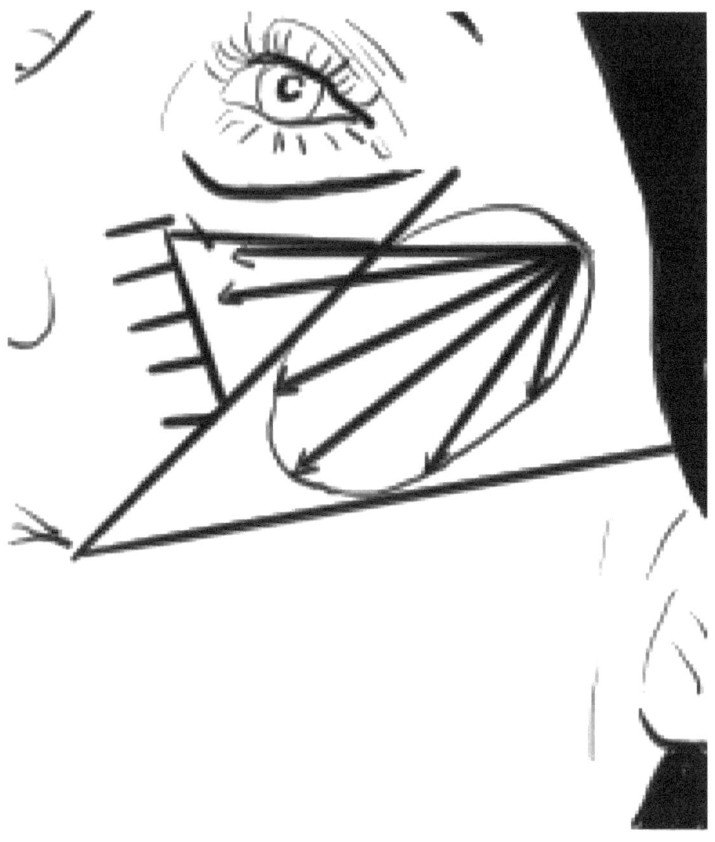

Secondly, after looking at this picture, you can evaluate the average amount of filler that may be inserted. Imagine, this area was injected with a vector technic. What happened with your nasolabial folds? Are they disappearing? What about the bags or hollows under your eyes? Do they look better? Is your face lifted after a volume of product is injected? One syringe is considered a minimum to inject within the middle third of one's face. If you are happy with the results the way they are, the injections may be complete. If you would like more noticeable results, additional injections can be done immediately or two weeks later, when 30% of the results will be noticeable.

We rarely inject directly into the nasolabial folds, as we previously did a decade before. The reason for changing this approach was common sense. When you put your fingers on the most prominent part of your cheekbones and lift them upwards, you will see that your nasolabial folds greatly disappear.

Using your phone, take a photo of your profile, please. Like this:

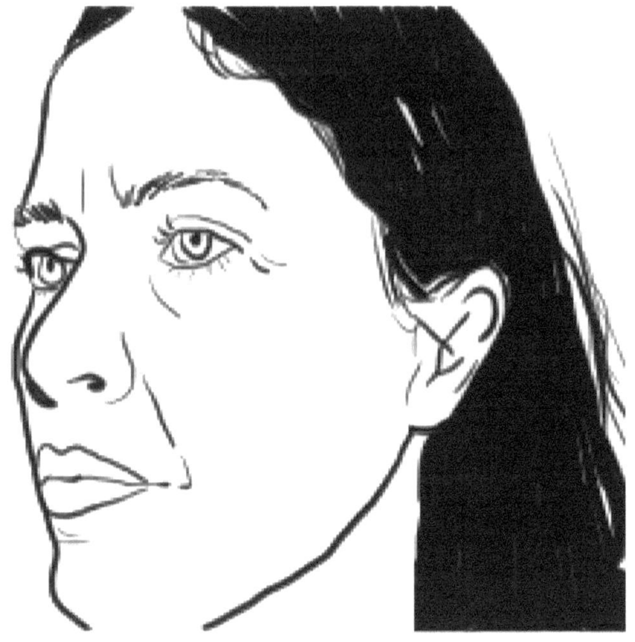

Now put your fingers near your ear and pull on the skin. Under your fingers, you definitely will feel how much volume you lost. As you pull your skin out, you will see how your nasolabial folds are improving, and the marionette lines are disappearing. This result helps you understand that injecting certain amounts in this area achieves removing the folds from the nose to lips and gets rid of lines under the corners of your mouth. Consider from 0,3 syringe to 0,5 syringe each side. Pay attention: nobody will see these areas as if they were injected with fillers, but everybody will see your face become more oval and younger-looking.

Lower 1/3 of the Face

First of all, let's figure out the most common concerns in this area. There are the "smoker lines," or wrinkles around the mouth, and the marionette lines, which are the wrinkles or folds near the corner of the mouth. Many clients point out volume lost near the chin, changing shape of the chin, as well as the appearance of the jaw. Many people deny these changes, seeing only aging of the lips.

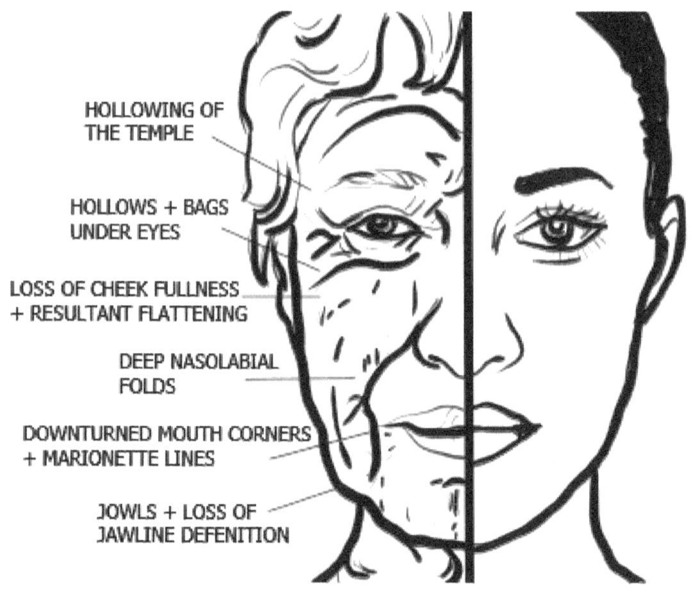

However, aging for the lower 1/3 of the face is much more complicated, and it is not only the lips that make a person look older. The changes in the bones, in the lower and upper jaws, make proportions different. Therefore, refilling the volume in the corners of the mouth and making the proportions fitted to a young face, as well as refilling the jaw angle, gives the lower face a younger appearance without jowls. Lip injection is the last step to make you look not only younger but natural.

The most complicated filler injections in this area involve refilling "smoker lines." A slight effect of bluish color sometimes appears under the eyes after injections. Clients complain of puffiness after fillers used in this area as well. It is not easy to balance the result and side effects. Moreover, it is impossible to get rid of these lines completely using fillers only. I would say that Mesotherapy/Bio- revitalization is a better solution. The difference is that this area is injected with non-cross-linked Hyaluronic acid. When you do this, it absolutely excludes the above-mentioned above side effects and pushes the skin to produce its own collagen to diminish the size of wrinkles.

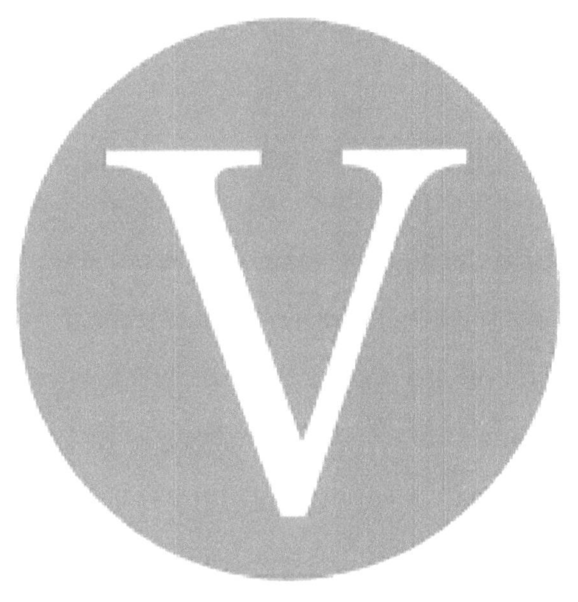

CHAPTER 8:
DOUBLE CHIN
AND JAWLINE

Reversing Time in the Lower Third of the Face

Not all clients asking about the correction of their jaw-lines have the deformative type of aging, which relates to an excessive fat deposit in the areas of the jaw and neck. After a certain age, people who experience a lack of fat in the face, see the imperfections of their jawline as well. It seems that after a certain age, everybody should think about defining the shape of the lower third of the face. The goal of defining the jawline logically includes several steps.

Sometimes I see clients who have significant double chins, insisting that they want to be injected by Botulinum toxin to get rid of jowls and make the jawline visible once again. They would most likely have read about the famous "Nefertiti Lift," and want to rely on only these treatments to get a perfect jawline (Levy, 2015). Unfortunately, this is impossible. It is necessary to get rid of fat in the chin area, and it is only after doing that, that we use injections of Botulinum toxins along with fillers to define the jawline more. Double chin is not the only problem related to fat deposits, but it represents complex, insufficient lymphatic drainage in the area, along with sagging skin, which relates to insufficient collagen support and spasming of muscles in the area. Removal of fat is possible using lipolytic injections, a product which resolves the fat. It is very popular to use a technology like Radio Frequency (RF) and simultaneously achieve the results of double chin fat removal and skin tightening.

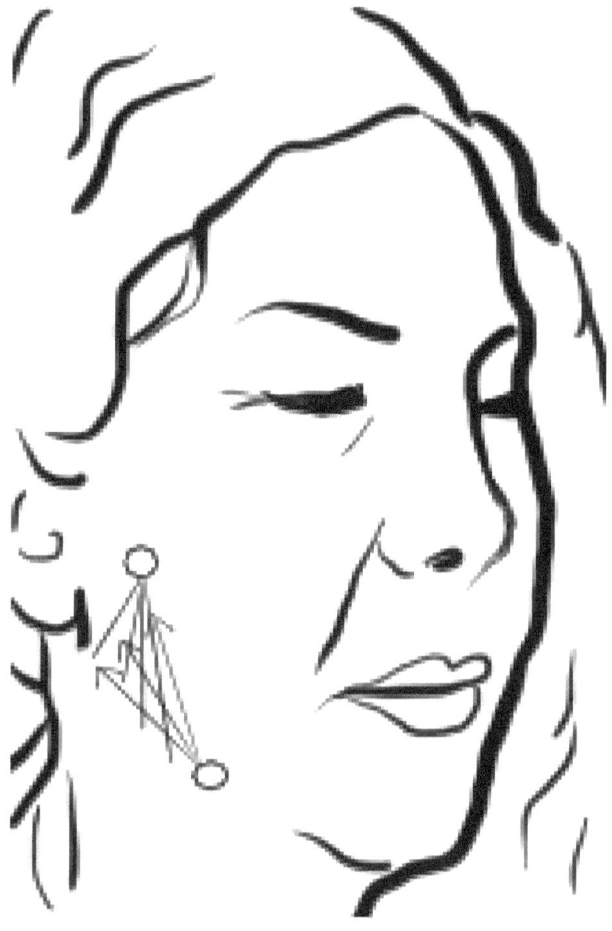

The removal of fat will often create excessive skin in the area where the fat once was. It is possible to reduce muscle tension and spread the amount of skin more evenly over relaxed muscles. Three points of neurotoxin injection on both sides of the face within the marionette wrinkle-causing muscles, as well as injections into the cords, decrease the tension of the muscles. This provides a more defined looking jawline within three weeks. Another way to handle excess skin is to pull it around on the frame on which it was built before. Fillers are used for this purpose. Fillers are injected into the middle part of the face, temple and chin areas, and the angles of the jaws. By injecting at the edges of the face, we stretch the skin like a tent. This "tent tension" helps to avoid unusually "prominent" cheekbones and makes a face look more natural. Skin tightening with RF or lasers is helpful when the goal is to reduce amounts of excess skin. To sum it up, the double chin removal program includes fat removal, muscle relaxation, lymphatic drainage, and skin tightening. It is clear that visible results can be reached only with the combined power of technology, Botulinum toxin, and fillers.

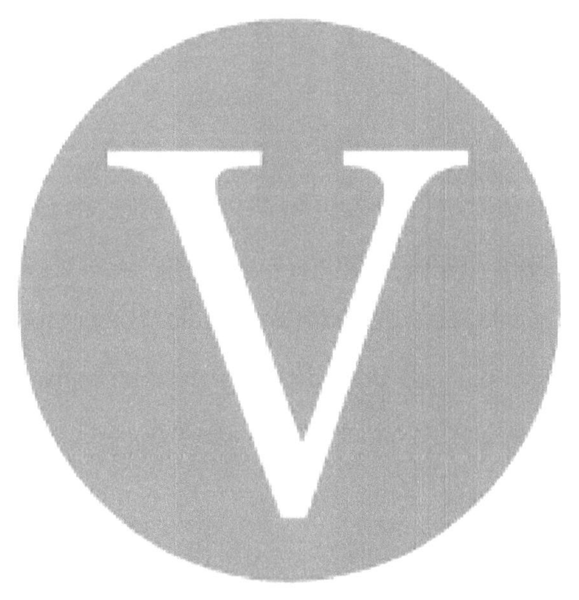

CHAPTER 9:
THE NATURAL LOOK

Why are Some People Overdone?

And why do some people look like overdone? People in the media who are judged by ordinary people, very often have visible signs of beauty injections on their faces. Their experience scares simple people. They come to the clinic with fear and prejudice toward injections. It is my goal to explain to them how everything is done in our field of medical aesthetics. I want to eliminate the fear and give them the tools to control the injections process.

There are several reasons, from my experience, why it becomes visible that "something was done," or "too much was done."

Some people are overdone because fillers were not in-jected in the right place. Most often we're looking to place injections in the middle central part of the face. Simply speaking, visible underlying cheekbones give a younger-looking appearance to young women. However, it creates a misunderstanding of age for mature women who are pretending to look younger. Curves on a face are markers of youth. Le Louarn explained that young people have curve-shaped muscles and fat pats under them. With age, we lose curves on a face, and cannot completely restore them. Therefore, visible underlying cheekbones on the face of a person, whose other features show aging, cannot look natural. To avoid this problem, it is recommended to inject in the right places, where face lost fat.

Reason number two why these two looks result is because the injections are not of the right volume. I see many people who have a concern that "it will be too much for them." These clients do not know how much is in a syringe and how much volume it can replace. To clarify the volume of a product, I would like you to think that five syringes are one tablespoon. How many syringes can be injected has to be decided on the volume which the client has lost. For example, four syringes for a 60-year-old lady is average. Whereas, some people at 60 who have spent years in a routine of skin tightening, laser resurfacing, or bio-revitalization injections don't need four syringes. They need maybe only two or even one syringe to replace the volume in some areas. So, the right amount is key for looking younger, but it should be considered for each exact case. The other concern is under-injections. These happen when the amount injected does not show the visible result of lifting. To avoid this problem, a consultation should be done before the injector's appointment, and the product and the amount necessary should be identified to produce a result of a younger-looking and rested appearance. In MedVspa, for example, we draw the injection map as well as give the client a consultation list where the minimum and a maximum number of syringes is recorded with the prices.

The next reason that optimum results are not achieved is due to not using the right type of injections. There is not much difference between the brands. So, each manufacturer only ever points out the strong-suits of the products, avoiding telling anyone the downfalls. The density and plasticity of the product play a significant role. For example, injecting in temple areas requires a product with a high level of plasticity. If a product of improper plasticity is chosen, other people will be able to see that something was injected. The area of the cheekbones requires structure. Therefore, a high-density product has to be injected. It's the responsibility of the injector to choose the right type of product. But remember, as it pertains to the temple, perioral area and all around the eyes, the specific density of the product needs to be known.

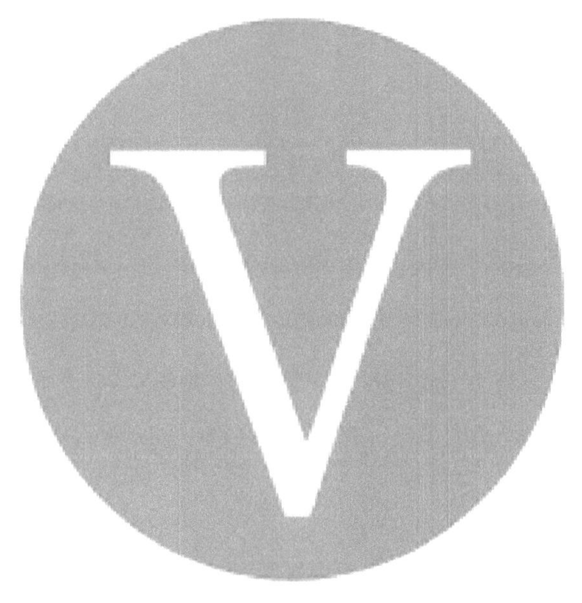

CHAPTER 10:
THE LONG-TERM GOALS

How Often Should I Have Injections?

It's very important what the manufacturers say about injections. In the case of fillers, manufacturers use them to confirm stability in the area for one or two years. We know that neurotoxin injections will last three to four months. Mesotherapy is recommended as a series of treatments for the timeframe of two weeks to one month between injections.

Let's talk about a young person who wants to prevent the appearance of strong wrinkles on the forehead, between the eyebrows. For such clients, the goal is to prevent the appearance of wrinkles by decreasing the strength of the facial muscles. To reach this goal, neurotoxin is injected into the muscles that are responsible for these wrinkles. We usually do injections of the Botulinum toxin in the area two or three times in intervals of three to six months. After individually assessing this person, we give her/him the right advice on how much product effectively weakens the muscles and how long of a period they may need to wait for further treatments.

The clients usually ask how long they will keep the lifted appearance that filler injections create. The length of the results may depend on many factors. The younger the client, the more effectivity is predicted. Postmenopausal age clients lose volume fast and therefore may need additional injections in six months. For such clients, one additional syringe is often enough.

Choose the practitioner who will be responsible for the improvement of your appearance within the next five years. Over-injection of fillers creates a problem for the injector in the future as well. For instance, after excess injections in the cheekbone area, excessive skin under the eyes can appear. Improper blockage of muscles around eyes caused by the Botulinum toxin can cause wrinkle formations in the inner corners of the eyes. If you commit to one practitioner long-term, he or she will be held responsible for such predictable side effects.

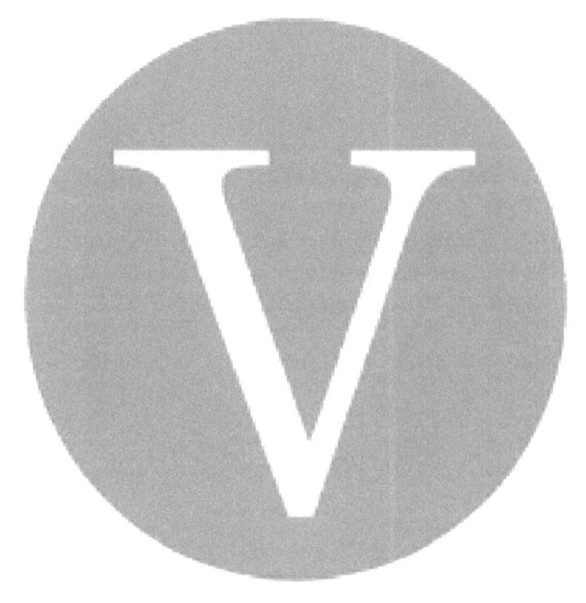

CHAPTER 11:
YOUR FACE'S SAFETY

What are the Criteria for Facial Injections?

According to the statistics, [HJ2] Botox is the most popular medical aesthetic treatment in the world, and only three percent of Botulinum toxin injections cause side effects. From my own experience, a worst-case scenario may be drooping eyelids that are easy to fix within two weeks.

In the case of filler injections, we are afraid of two things. Number one is trapping the vessel. That is why when the injection is done with a needle; we use a special test to see whether we are in a blood vessel or not. To avoid such complications, specialists often use cannulas. Cannulas look like very long needles, but they are not sharp. The length is usually five centimeters. We create a small hole and insert the cannula, maintaining absolute 100% assurance of not damaging any vessels. In addition, it's not painful for the client at all.

The second side effect is the affection of blood flow and lymph in the area of injections. This happens when more than 1/3 of the syringe is injected in one place. The result can be swelling or changing of the color of tissues within the area of injection. Usually, injections done with a needle cause this side effect.

To avoid such complications, it is recommended to use cannulas for injections while avoiding the over-injection of product into one area.

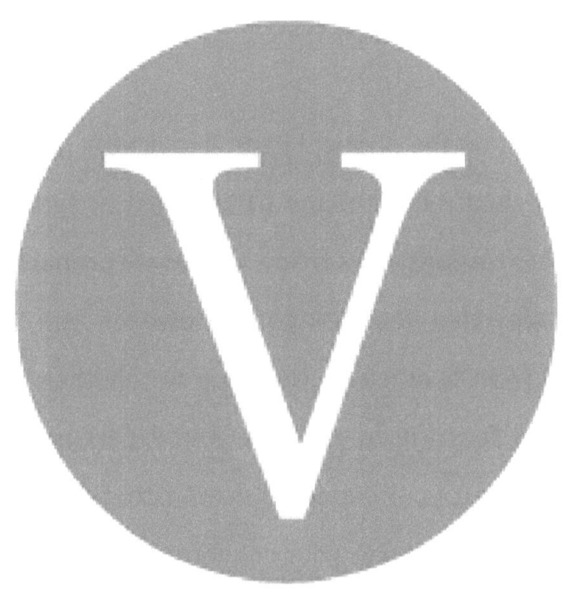

CHAPTER 12:
START FROM THE CONSULTATION

What Can You Expect?

Sometimes on the phone, I hear "I look very good at 64. I do not think I need many treatments, or syringes, or units." My response is as follows: "You are probably right. I am happy that you look good. However, you NEED a CONSULTATION at least." Next, we sit together; you address your concerns to us; share your experience with us and talk about your expectations. Aesthetic is a part of medicine. We evaluate your concerns from the prism of skin aging physiology and anatomy. We will support your realistic expectations and will be responsible for the promised result. We start from the assessment, then beginning to write a treatment plan for you. Exactly for you, because medically speaking, people age differently. The treatment plan is usually divided up by steps and includes: Step 1: Correction of wrinkles related to facial expressions. Injections of the Botulinum toxin relax muscles and wrinkles disappear. These injections work well in the areas between the eyebrows, on forehead lines, and on the upper lip. Botulinum toxin starts working within a time period of three days to two weeks. The effect will be relaxed muscles and lifted areas. The length of the effect is three to six months.

Step 2: Correction of wrinkles and folds. Injection of fillers, usually cross-linked Hyaluronic Acid, improves volume, and significantly diminishes the depth of wrinkles. Side effects of these injections include possible bruising, redness, and swelling.

Step 3: Improvement of the texture of skin and hydration in the areas of the face, neck, décolleté, and hands.

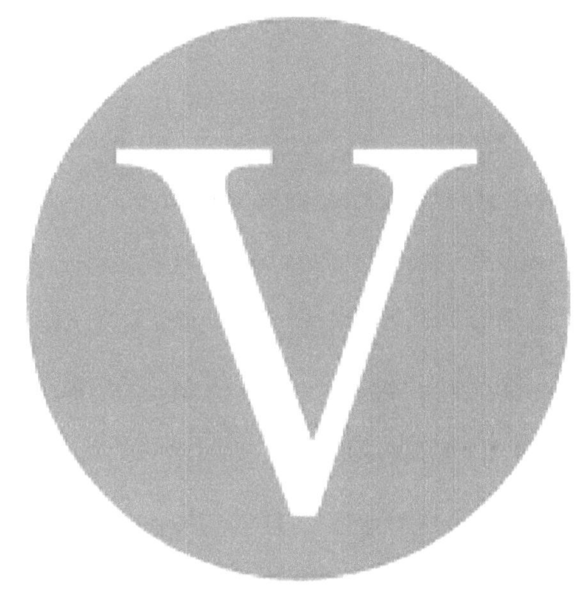

CHAPTER 13:
THE INJECTION CARD

What Your Injector Needs to Know

Before any injections, it is necessary to evaluate the aging type. There are four types, as follows;

Sagging skin type: These people are mostly Europeans with pale, thin skin. With age, the skin gets covered by many shallow wrinkles caused by changes in the collagen structure and insufficient deep skin hydration.

Tired type of aging representatives do not look good because of signs of fatigue on their faces. They complain about drooping eyelids, angular eyes that make them appear depressed, and nasolabial folds.

Deformative type representatives show the main sign of aging as gravitational ptosis. Ptosis is a result of redeposition of the fat. Redeposition of the fat from the middle third to the lower third of the face makes the jawline almost invisible, and a double chin replaces the line.

In the Muscular type of aging, the muscles of the face are very strong. Wrinkles and folds in the areas of the upper and lower eyelids, drooping corners of the lips, and nasolabial folds, all appear as signs of aging. Most of the people who age showing the muscular skin type see dark spots and discoloration on their faces in their early forties.

The second important thing to understand is the pattern of facial expressions, which is genetically determined. Identifying the pattern of facial expressions within the mother enables a specialist to predict wrinkles that could appear in the future. For example, if the client answers that she has forehead wrinkles from her 20s and that her mom has deep lines in this area as well after the evaluation of such data, it is better to make injections of the Botulinum toxin with the goal to prevent unwanted facial expression patterns and the appearance of deep wrinkles.

The third determining factor of aging is the type of facial muscle activity and the condition of the muscles themselves. This group of clients will note of strong facial muscles, and they will want relaxation to get rid of wrinkles. Usually, they are representatives of a younger age group. When the muscles are strong and balanced (without visible asymmetry), we easily relax them by using Botulinum toxin. However, after a certain age, muscular balance may not quite be what it once was. This means that those parts of the muscles are more active in a chronic hypertonic condition. You see people with deep lines between eyebrows or on their foreheads. These people cannot relax these muscles even when they're at rest and not trying to express any emotions. In addition, men and women have a different type of facial muscle activity as well as muscle strength. Consequently, dosages and injection points are different for them.

Lastly, we need to know the amount of volume lost by the client, so we are able to restore said volume.

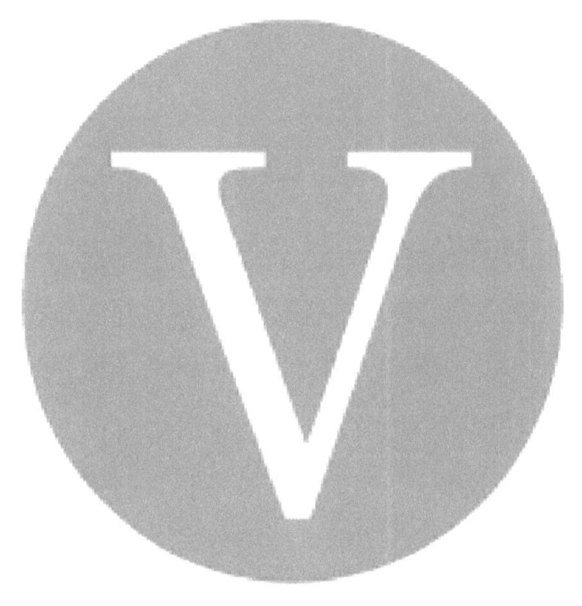

CHAPTER 14:
TREATMENT OF AGING ON THE FOREHEAD

What Botulinum Toxin can do for the Forehead

There are several patterns of forehead movements. The injection card is developed according to these patterns, which means the injector must keep in mind the different forms of forehead muscle contractions. The number of injection sites is based on the goals we would like to reach. If the goal is complete muscle relaxation, four injection sites are performed. However, if the goal is more sophisticated and includes a balance of lifting and muscle relaxation, many injections will be performed. Usually, the number of injection sites does not exceed[HJ8]

Considering the fact, that in a case of disabling forehead muscles exclusively, the strength of the forehead could be transferred to the group of muscles between the eyebrows. Injections between the eye brows are then performed at the same time. A smaller dosage is used for the area between the eyebrows if the aim is to relax forehead muscles exclusively.

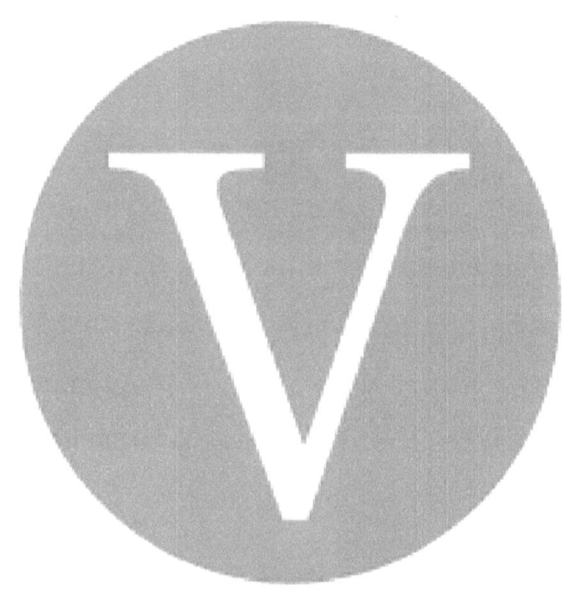

CHAPTER 15:
THE HATED "ELEVENTH"

How do You Get Rid of the Frown Lines?

Strong muscles between eyebrows are responsible for the firm "eleventh" appearance. Everybody wants to get rid of these lines in the center of the face. Sometimes it is impossible to remove them completely. Therefore, the earlier we decrease the strength of these muscles, the less of a chance you have to develop "eleventh" permanently.

Before we discover your exact eyebrow movement pattern, please pay attention to your eyebrows when you are completely relaxed. Do they have a form of an arch, or are they more horizontal? Start frowning. Do you see your eyebrows coming together or going down? When you express animosity, do you see that the only areas expressing this emotion are the eyebrows, nose, forehead, and eyes as well?

There are different eyebrow pattern movements. Understanding these movement patterns helps you to understand how many points you will need when being

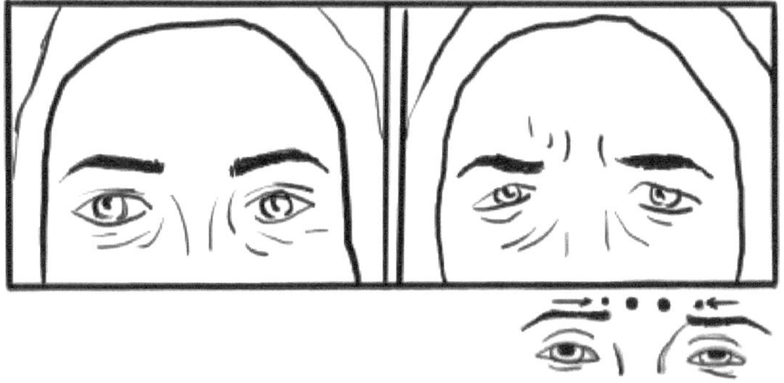

injected and what's going to be the pattern of injection. Moreover, I will help you to understand your face better when it comes to the aging process. Let's start!

ARROW PATTERN

Please frown. Look at the movements of your eyebrows. Do your eyebrows move horizontally, resembling a converting arrow? Is there any depression at the eyebrow level? If so, you are a representative of the "Converting Arrow pattern." This pattern is the second most common in men and the third most common in women. Injections will need 3 -5 points in the area between eyebrows. The goal for these injections is to relax the "arrows" which create wrinkles and give the face an angry appearance.

U-PATTERN

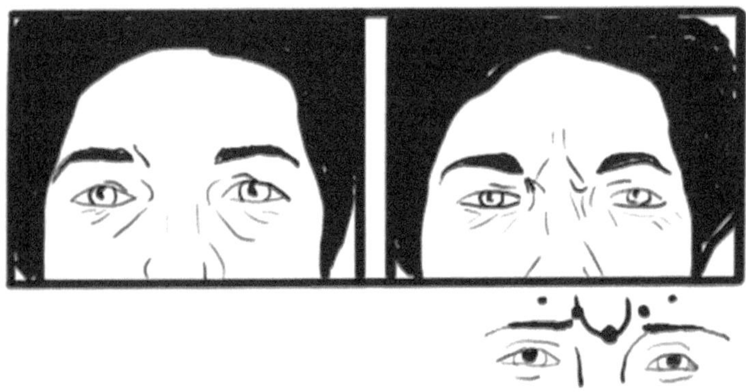

The U-PATTERN is the most common glabella movement, and it resembles a U-letter. Please look at the mirror without any movement. Does your eyebrow shape resemble an arch? Now please frown and pay attention to the depression appearing between your eyebrows while frowning. Do you see a similarity with the letter U? If yes, you are struggling with the same issue as 32% of the population. Moreover, this pattern of movement is the most common among women. You will probably be injected in five sites, and a standard dosage of neurotoxin will be used on you.

V-PATTERN

A V-PATTERN occurs when you're relaxed, and your eyebrows are more rectified and lower. If that is the case, you will probably see the V-way of eyebrow frowning. People who have the

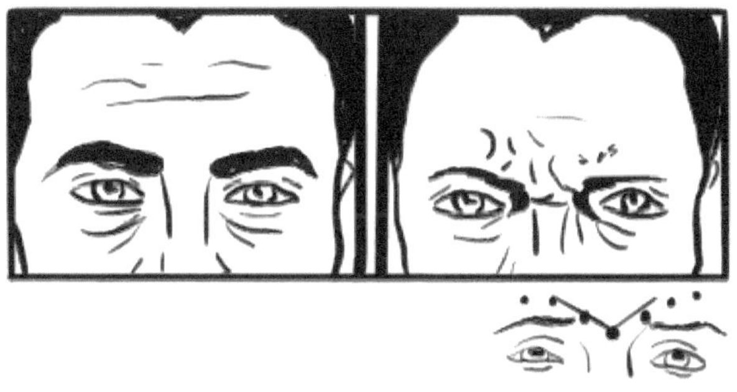

V-pattern of this movement have stronger muscles between the eyebrows. Therefore, they need a higher dosage of neurotoxin to relax these muscles. When injecting the neurotoxin, we don't want the product to migrate. We inject the smallest dose possible to the target muscles with the goal to decrease the movement range exclusively in these muscles. Consequently, if a muscle is strong and needs a higher dosage to be relaxed, the injection sites will be divided. Therefore, expect seven injection points and a higher dosage for real muscle relaxation. This pattern of movement is second among women and first in the male population.

OMEGA PATTERN

Does your frowning resemble the Greek letter Omega? When

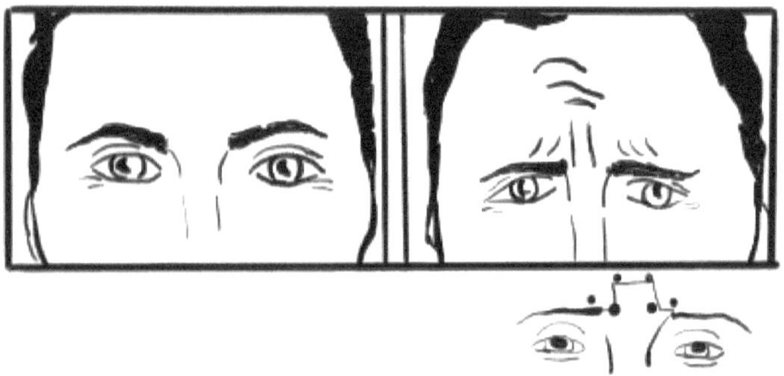

pretending to be angry, do you see the movement of the forehead muscles under the heads of the eyebrows, and muscles in the inner part of the eye? If so, you are fairly unique as only 10% of the population frown this way. Expect three to five injection sites in the areas of the eyebrows and forehead muscles.

INVERTED OMEGA PATTERN

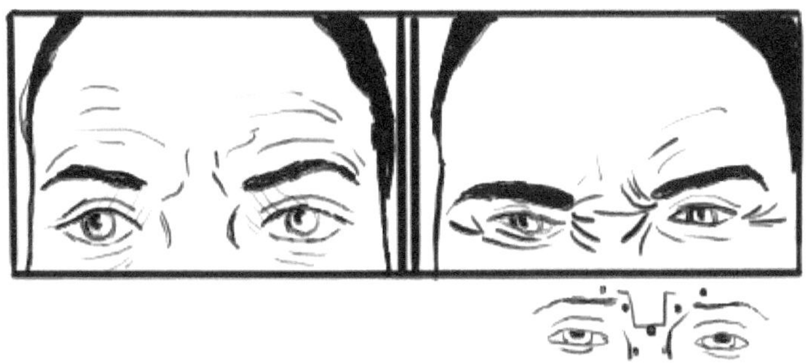

A lot of muscles help you to express anger. Not only the muscles between the eyebrows, but also small muscles in the inner corner of the eyes, as well as nasals muscles (your nose is moving when you're speaking...). Expect injections between the eyebrows and in the nose. We have to block all muscles' otherwise, the strength of one muscle will be transformed to others inside the conglomerate.

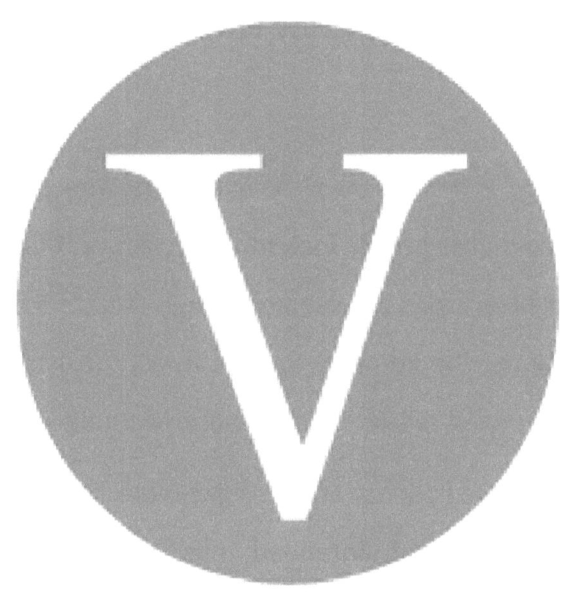

CHAPTER 16:
AN EYE OPENER

Open Eyes and Eyebrow Lifting
with Injections

Everybody wants to lift their eyebrows. The open eye look only makes people look more attractive. Moreover, the lack of wrinkles between eyebrows creates a friendly appearance. The lifting of the eyebrows consists of two parts: forehead relaxation and eyebrow lifting.

The majority of clients after 50 get more benefits from face lifting through forehead muscle relaxation, and much less from full muscle block. The block of forehead muscles runs the risk of the eyebrows falling. As the forehead muscle thins with age, an increasingly smaller number of units can be a reason for eyebrows falling. In addition, after a certain age, people use their eyebrows and forehead to keep their eyes wide open. Excessive relaxation of the forehead muscle will not allow it to be used to lift the eyebrows. To avoid this situation, neurotoxin injections for forehead lifting are usually done about two weeks after the injections into the area between the eyebrows. A smaller dosage is recommended for aging clients. They cannot expect complete forehead muscle blockage because of the factors listed above. When the neurotoxin is injected in the 6-8-point pattern, it is expected that the forehead will not freeze but will become more relaxed and lifted. However, it is also expected that the effects of the Botulinum toxin lifting pattern will not be as permanent as the effect of injections done in the 4-point pattern, which predictably show a more relaxed appearance.

Many years of experience dealing with aging clients, especially Europeans, brings a lot of corrections into classic injection recommendations as well.

There are different technics for injections in the area around the eyes. We have a certain dosage, recommended by the manufacturers for injections in this area. Manufacturers advise injecting in three sites for each eye. It works very well for young people who don't have a hernia and who don't suffer from eye swelling. However, other factors are involved when we're thinking about Botulinum toxin injections in the area around the eyes. Let's take a look at some of them.

Many people have a specific way of smiling. They smile more with their cheeks than their eyes. The classic technic of injections for this group of clients is to stop the moving up of cheekbones and inhibit the creation of additional wrinkles around the eyes. The wrinkles form in this manner because other muscles, called synergists, are involved in smiling. One more example is when a client is smiling with their nose. A complete blockage of the muscle around the eye reinforces the strength of the nose muscles. For an aging group of clients, smiling can show wrinkles spreading from the eyes to the cheekbones.

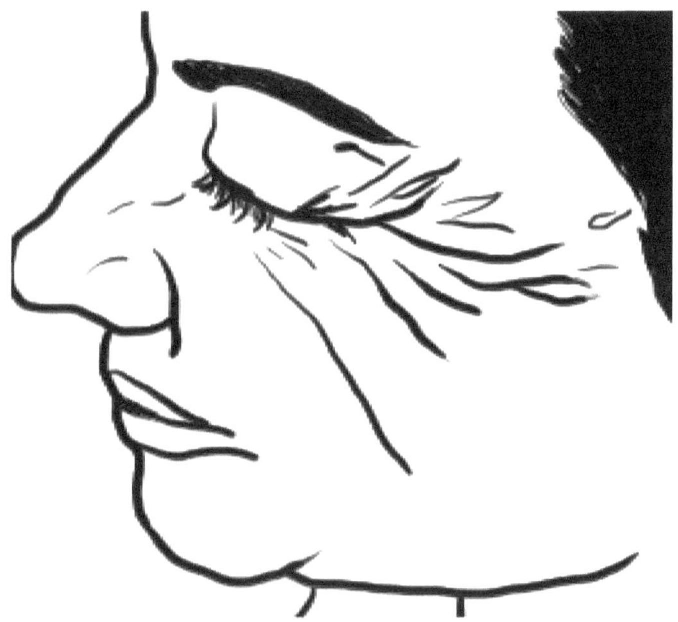

Moreover, the drainage function of this periorbital area is changing as the consequence of aging; therefore, people complain about eye swelling more often. All of these factors should be considered before injections.

Specifically, in this area, we have to think more about injection technics and less about dosage. We use a technic called mesotoxin instead of the classic recommendation in many cases. The goal is to relax the skin rather than muscles.

To sum up. The classical 3-point technique is effective for young people exclusively. Clients who smile with their cheekbones and aging clients have to be injected using the special "mesotoxin" technique.

The Meso Botox technique means that many sites of injections will be delivered to the skin. Injections are so superficial that white bumps become visible immediately. The bumps disappear within 5-10 minutes. The effect shows faster. When smiling, some skin movements are less pronounced. The effect is very natural but lasts shorter. The "open eye" technique was offered by Korean specialists several years ago. It consists of three injection sites being performed very close to the eyelid margin. A numbing cream is recommended before these injections. The open eye technique is recommended for people who squint while focusing their eyes.

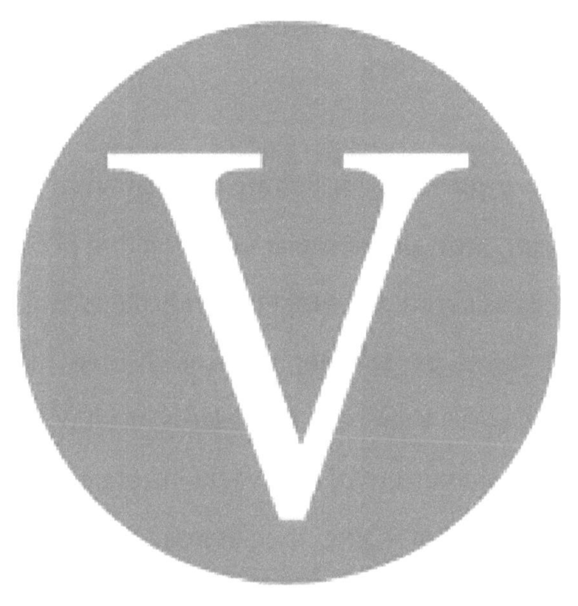

CHAPTER 17:
LIPS – THE MOST
"FEARFUL" AREA

Why You Can't Look Complete without Lip Fillers

Injections involving aging lips are different in comparison to younger ones. Under the assumption that proper protocol is considered and practiced, ridiculous looking fillers will never be another stressor. People may look ridiculous when they have had excess injections. That is why we have a pattern of two weeks in between injection sessions. We inject some, then assess the person within two weeks. If we feel it's necessary, we'll add more syringes into the process. If unnecessary, clients may skip getting more.

When we inject, we use the "criteria for beautiful lips." The lip line should be horizontal. Lips end at the two parallel lines between the pupils. The lower lip looks bigger and fuller than upper.

The length of the ideal nose is around 5 cm, and it's located in the exact midway space between the pupils. The nasolabial fold is barely visible, and the cupidone arch, philtrum columns and curves of the upper and lower lips are clear. These criteria are based on the research of Fabio Meneghini, a Clinical Facial Analysis, (Springer, 2005).

This is especially important to remember working with aging clients. They have major concerns over their lips losing volume. By adding volume and opening up the lip corners, it is possible to make the mouth bigger than 50 mm. Therefore, for some aging clients, it is better not to lift up the lip corners to make the lips look more attractive and natural. The second criteria are the nasolabial folds. We have to diminish them to see the area surrounding the lips looking younger. However, nasolabial folds are a sign of structural aging and are very often a consequence of the face dropping down in the middle. You can easily check this when you put your fingers in the prominent parts of the cheekbones and try to lift up the skin slightly. Do you see that this lift is improving the appearance of the nasolabial folds? If yes, you know that the solution is to correct the middle one-third of the face with fillers.

The volume of the lower lip is supposed to be bigger compared to the upper. The weight of the upper lip being bigger than the lower is the criteria for young lips.

In Profile:

1. The most prominent point of the lower lip is slightly shifted outward.

2. The upper lip in the profile is showing a slight bulge.

3. The Ricket's line is 4mm from the upper lip and 2mm from the lower lip.

4. The lower lip is plumper than the upper lip.

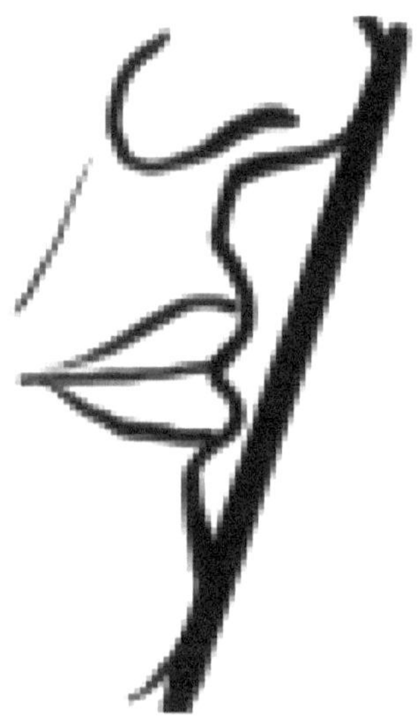

What are the results of lip correction? You can expect that after the correction the lower lip is larger than the upper, proportional to your actual lip shape. The lips will have a sharper contour. The most prominent point of the lower lip will be slightly shifted outward. The upper lip in profile will be showing a slight bulge (you will enjoy your profile pictures more). Ideally, the nasolabial fold will be less visible.

In my practice, I start lip injections for clients after 45 with a very small amount, 0,3 cc, using the insulin syringe. I do it because almost all clients are really scared to have weird, big lips as a result of getting lip fillers. Two weeks afterward, I invite them for the follow-up appointment and ask them how they look and how they feel. Almost all clients like the new appearance of their lips very much. Really, they are the only ones seeing the difference in lip shape and enjoying the brighter color.

Ninety percent of clients become braver after a small injection and insist on injecting more. This very small touch can dramatically change their self-acceptance.

I am happy about my clients' changes, however aging lips and young lips have different criteria when it comes to beauty; therefore, they need to be injected in a different way to look natural.

Let's talk about that. Young Lips need correction when they are asymmetrical when the volume of the upper lip is significantly smaller than the lower, when lips are thin or small compared to the face and when they do not have a clean contour. Young lips are injected with the goal of adding volume, contouring, and turning them out or lifting them. However, only young lips will look sexy when the upper lip is wider compared to the lower. Like this:

Aged Lips require correction to add volume and symmetry, to get rid of lip wrinkles, and to diminish the marionette lines.

Working with lip contour is different for young and aging lips. For aging lips, we have to consider that aging skin over the upper lip does not have the density, of young skin. Therefore, lip contour injections require specificity. The migration of the product into the empty upper lip space is considered. Therefore, the amount and density of the product is important. I see people who have an "upper double lip" shape because of product migration.

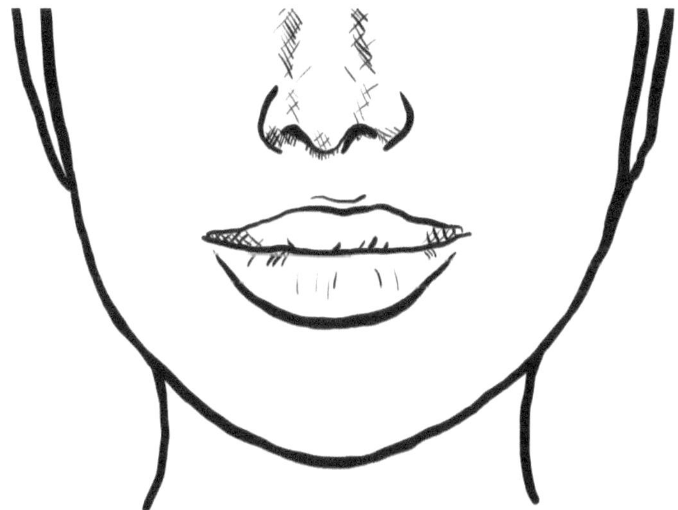

Last generation products, when injected with a smaller amount using a specific technique, leads to a decrease in the chance of product migration significantly. A small amount of filler, injected with the insulin syringe, make lips look plumper and fuller, without wrinkles, more symmetrical, and desirably natural.

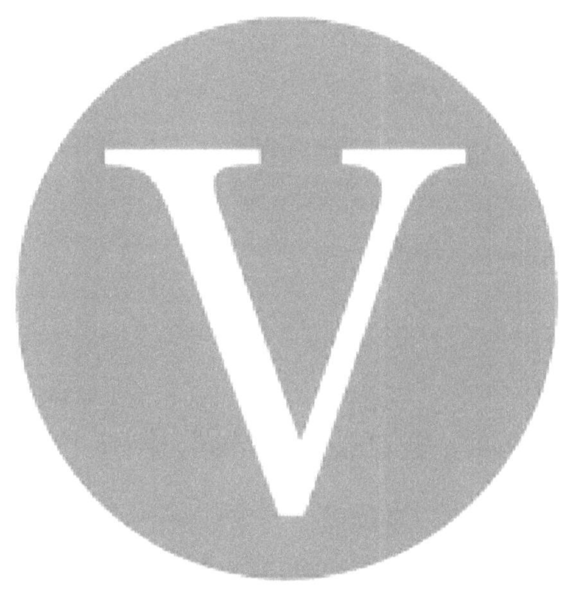

CHAPTER 18:
AFTERWORD

Why This Matters

Honestly, I like to do injections. It's the fastest way to change someone's appearance and to make the client happy with how they look.

When a client who is 55 comes for a treatment, she is looking to replace volume. What she sees is probably sagging skin, and a lot of deep wrinkles on her forehead or nasolabial folds. We consider her condition from both the structural and tissue aging perspective. The best way to restore her volume is by using fillers. We need to subdue her strong muscles and to give her face a relaxed and calm appearance. After that, it is much easier to decrease the amount of excess skin and fix skin discoloration, texture, and density. We have to build a plan from the beginning to target all the problematic areas. After completing said program, the client should walk away (not completely, don't forget occasional maintenance) with vibrant, good-looking skin, and a lifted face without wrinkles or a double chin.

Because of injections, I have many happy guests. This gives me a sense of happiness, as well. That is why I'm traveling around the world nonstop learning about new products and techniques in the field of injections. I do this to bring new techniques and technologies back to my Canadian market and to change the lives of people who come seeking aging remedies.

REFERENCES

1. De Maio M, Rzany B. Patient selection. In: De Maio M, Rzany B, editors. *Botulinum Toxin in Aesthetic Medicine*. Berlin: Springer; 2007:11–19

2. De Maio, M. (2018). Myomodulation with injectable fillers: An innovative approach to addressing facial muscle movement. *Aesthetic plastic surgery, 42*(3), 798-814.

3. E. R., MD, & Kadunc, B. V., MD, PhD. (2012, July). *Glabellar Contraction Patterns: A Tool t Optimize Botulinum Toxin Treatment* [PDF]. DERMATOLOGIC SURGERY.

4. Le Louran, C., MD. (2007). Face Recurve. Retrieved 2019, from http://www.lelouarn.net/en/face-recurve

5. Levy, P. M. (2015). Neurotoxins: current concepts in cosmetic use on the face and neck—jawline contouring/platysma bands/necklace lines. *Plastic and reconstructive surgery, 136*(5S), 80S-83S.

ABOUT THE AUTHOR

Hello, my name is Marina Vashkevich.

I am a dermatologist in Belarus, a registered nurse (RN) in Canada and the USA, and the founder of MedVspa clinics in Europe, the United States, and Canada.

I created these clinics because I was seeing the same approach and the same technology being used everywhere to treat skin ailments.

Over my years of experience, I discovered that there was more to rejuvenating the skin than using one technology.

So, I created a unique combination of treatment protocols never seen in the industry before with maximum results to make my patients years younger. Through my experience as a dermatologist and an international speaker at aesthetic-medicine conferences, I have developed my own view on the aging process.

My decision to be an aesthetic dermatologist was unexpected for my colleagues and family. After graduating from medical school in Belarus, I worked as a psychiatrist for 15 years, rehabilitating drug-addicted teenagers.

Every medical doctor who has had the experience of working with drug-addicted teenagers will confirm that emotionally you won't be able to stay in this field for long. It was unbearable watching, every day, how amazing, beautiful people passed away due to an overdose; how twins, the only sons of their mother, were sent to prison for many years because they were drug dealers; and how parents wishing their drug-addicted children would die because they were not able to bear seeing how horrible their children were becoming. After 15 years, I needed a change and decided I wanted to start helping people in other ways.

My unhappy circumstances created a physical problem. I became sick and went through a series of back surgeries. Recovery was horrible with lots of pain and 100 percent dependency on the people around me. It was impossible to sit on a chair or even lift my leg up onto a step. The three months that I spent in different hospitals gave me the time to think about what I should next in life. This became a priceless treasure for me. I finally answered this question; I wanted to be an aesthetic dermatologist for my 20th year as a doctor. It was now or never! Realizing this helped me to recover.

My dermatology residency was a thousand kilometers from my home city. I was not able to sit properly, carry something that weighed more than six pounds, or walk a thousand steps, and my brain was impaired by painkillers, but I was the happiest I had been. It seems that struggle followed me twelve hours per day. I took the extended program. I learned, watched, and asked questions. I remember being hungry for knowledge about the skin, dermatology, creams, technologies, fillers, and so on. This continued for three years. I never had a free weekend or time to read for fun or watch movies. The most interesting things to read for me were scientific dermatology books and magazines. I remember my first job; I asked everyone everything, and like a sponge, I absorbed everyone's knowledge and experience. People shared generously, and I looked at them with such hungry but sparkling eyes, asking for knowledge.

One year later, while participating in a dermatology class discussion, I started to answer the doctors' questions instead of them answering mine. Immediately, I was recruited by Viora, a world leader and manufacturer of skin-care technology systems in the United States and Europe, and was offered a contract for the clinical trials of their new system, which at the time was called Reaction. I was happy and excited. It predetermined my next step. I opened my own practice and started to take clients, work with them directly, evaluate results, optimize protocols, and build new protocols for the treatments, combining technologies, injections, and chemical peels. I have seen wrinkles disappear, faces lifted, and skin restored to its youthful glow. It was a new found happiness to make people's dreams a reality!

My experience and success became known by many of my colleagues around the world, and as a result, I was invited to conferences as a speaker in Asia, the Middle

East, Europe, and Russia. I talked about my hands-on experience in treating acne, getting rid of wrinkles and double chins, performing eye lifts, and shrinking excess skin after extreme weight loss. I combined technologies and built my own protocols.

But it was not enough. North America lured me in with its outstanding medical experience. I left my Belarus clinic in the hands of one of my top practitioners and moved my family to Canada.

I started my business eight months after coming to Canada, and a year later, I opened a location in the United States.

My clients inspired me not only to open a clinic in Bloor-Yorkville, Toronto but also to write a book. All that you find in this book is my hands-on international experience. It is my consultation approach—everything that I discuss with the client during the consultation. These are my conclusions, based on the most up-to-date knowledge in the field of international aesthetic medicine.

It is never too late to start something from the beginning, whatever your age. It is never too late to seize your passion and, for once in your life, do something that you have always dreamed about doing.

I am happy to present this book to you. I want to share my happiness with the results that I see. I want you to stop spending hours searching the Internet and reading about aging, your neck, and cellulite. I explain everything to you the way I do to my clients. What you will discover in this book will save you time and money and give you a new perspective on life. You can look years younger; there are combinations of technologies and treatments that can help, and I will show you how. I am a very happy person now, and I am happy that I found the time, stopped, looked around, and shared everything that I know with you to make you happier.

Welcome to the magic of aesthetic medicine!

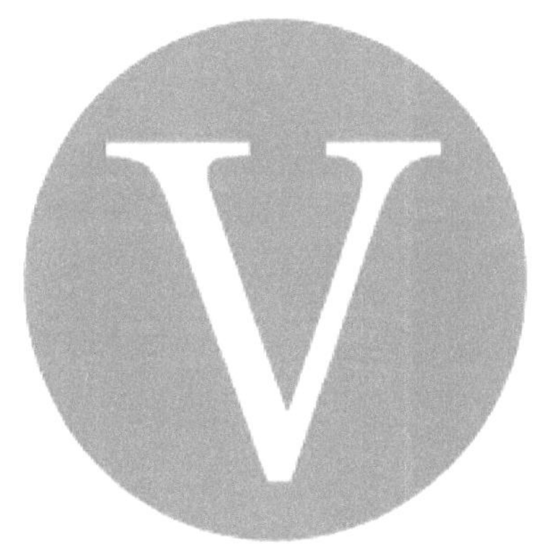

www.MedVSpa.com

Med V Spa
Toronto, Canada

Phone: (647) 460-4585